Hanen DHOUIB
Wièm BEN AMAR
Samir MAATOUG

Regulatory and ethical aspects of telemedicine

Hanen DHOUIB
Wièm BEN AMAR
Samir MAATOUG

Regulatory and ethical aspects of telemedicine

telemedicine: legal and ethical aspects

ScienciaScripts

Imprint
Any brand names and product names mentioned in this book are subject to trademark, brand or patent protection and are trademarks or registered trademarks of their respective holders. The use of brand names, product names, common names, trade names, product descriptions etc. even without a particular marking in this work is in no way to be construed to mean that such names may be regarded as unrestricted in respect of trademark and brand protection legislation and could thus be used by anyone.

Cover image: www.ingimage.com

This book is a translation from the original published under ISBN 978-620-2-54927-1.

Publisher:
Sciencia Scripts
is a trademark of
International Book Market Service Ltd., member of OmniScriptum Publishing Group
17 Meldrum Street, Beau Bassin 71504, Mauritius
Printed at: see last page
ISBN: 978-620-3-20940-2

TABLE OF CONTENTS

LIST OF ABBREVIATIONS

STROKE   : Stroke

CDM   : Code of Medical Ethics

CNOM   : National Council of the Order of Physicians

CPT   : Tunisian Penal Code

DMI   : Computerized Medical Record

EHPAD   : Etablissement d'hébergement pour personnes âgées dépendantes (Nursing home for dependent elderly people)

HIPPA   : Health Insurance Portability and Accountability Act

INDPP   : National Data Protection Authority

WHO   World Health Organization

ICT   Information and Communication Technologies

LIST OF FIGURES

LIST OF TABLES

Introduction

Faced with a rapidly changing environment, the Tunisian healthcare system is in perpetual transformation due to changing healthcare needs and the emergence of new technologies. Nowadays, digital tools, particularly through connected objects or devices, measure, analyze, store and sometimes share our health data. These digital technologies applied to health care cover the field of e-health or telehealth and offer new possibilities of access to care, new fields in the organization of care [1,2]. The applications of telehealth are broad, ranging from diagnostic or therapeutic telemedicine to "informative" or medico-social telemedicine [3].

Telemedicine is increasingly emerging as a relevant solution to meet the challenges facing healthcare systems, such as changing medical demographics, territorial inequalities in access to care, the rising prevalence of chronic diseases and the aging of the population. However, despite all these considerable advances and progress for humanity, telehealth can be the source of numerous conflicts and practical, ethical and legal difficulties such as: transparency, medical secrecy, protection of patients' personal medical data and respect for privacy [4]. In Tunisia, as in many countries, there are laws to protect our health data and respect their confidentiality, however, it is useful to study the applicability of these laws to new health technologies and the degree to which they respect patient rights and ethical principles.

The objectives of this work are :

- To study the legal framework of telemedicine in Tunisia in the light of comparative law.
- Analyze the ethical problems posed by new information and communication technologies used in the health field.

Materials and methods

1. DEFINITIONS :

Videoconferencing or videoconferencing is an interactive process, combining audiovisual, computer and telecommunications technologies, through which people at remote sites can, in real time, see each other, dialogue and exchange written or audio documents.

Tele-assistance is defined as a medical act performed by a physician when he or she remotely assists another physician or health professional in performing a medical or surgical procedure.

2. TYPE OF STUDY AND TARGET POPULATION :

We conducted a survey among doctors practicing at CHU Habib BOURGUIBA in Sfax, CHU Charles NICOLLE and Salah AZAIEZ in Tunis.

- Inclusion Criteria :

All surgical specialty physicians, regardless of rank.

- Exclusion Criteria :

Physicians who refused to answer the questionnaire.

3. METHODOLOGY :

We designed a 16-item questionnaire with simple-choice questions (Appendix 1):

- A first part collecting information on participant characteristics (gender, age, specialty, grade).
- A second part inviting them to describe their experience with videoconferencing.
- A third part concerning their views on the benefits of telehealth, as well as its ethical and legal issues.

We sent the questionnaire by email, using google Forms.

The questionnaire was only available on the internet. Participants were encouraged to answer it by an e-mail that provided the link to access the questionnaire. The estimated time required to complete the questionnaire was 10 minutes.

4. DATA ENTRY AND ANALYSIS :

The data was captured and analyzed using SPSS 24.0 software.

Quantitative variables were described using means, medians, standard deviation, and limits.

Qualitative variables were described using proportions.

Results

Of the 89 physicians to whom we sent the form, 39 agreed to respond, for a participation rate of 43.8%.

1.PERSONAL DATA OF THE PARTICIPATING DOCTORS :

1.1 Gender Distribution of the Study Population :

Most participants were male as shown in Figure 1.

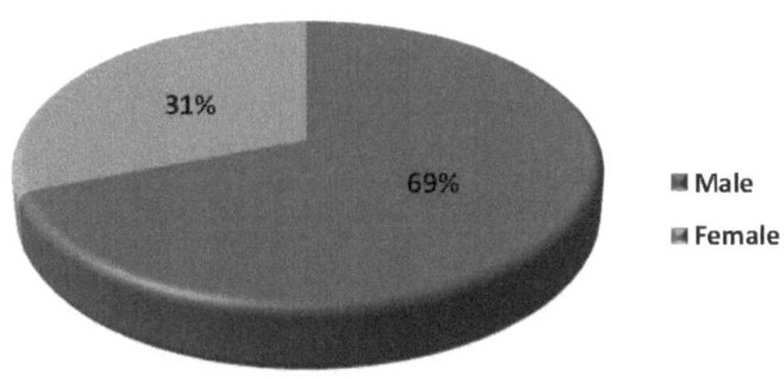

Figure 1: Gender Distribution of the Study Population

1.2 Age Distribution of the Study Population :

The median age of participants was 33 years (percentiles: 30-36 years) with extremes of 27 and 58 years.

1.3. Distribution of the study population by specialty :

Among the physicians who responded to our questionnaire, visceral surgeons were in the majority (38.5% of cases). (Figure 2)

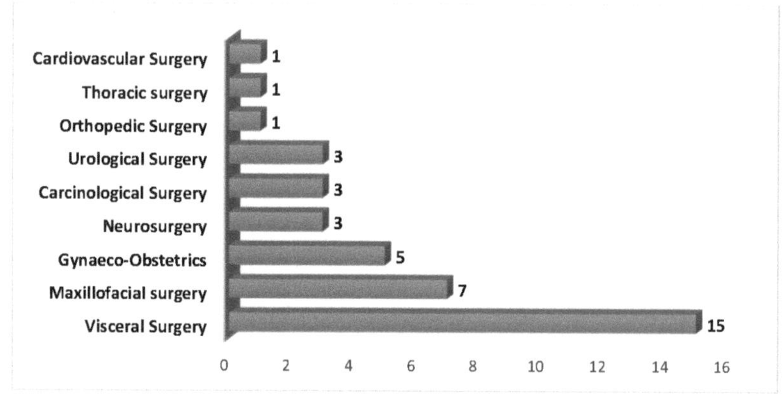

Figure 2: Distribution of Study Population by Specialty

1.4. Distribution of the study population by grade :

Resident physicians are the most represented category in 48.7% of cases, followed by teaching hospital assistants in 23.1% of cases, as shown in Figure 3.

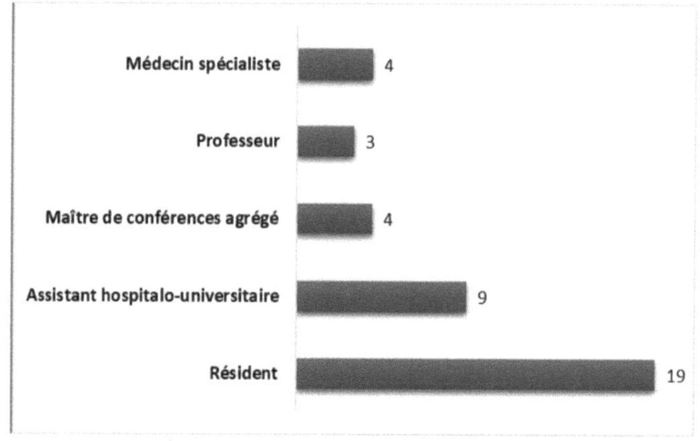

Figure 3: Distribution of Study Population by Grade

2. DATA RELATING TO THE CONCEPT OF TELE-MEDICAL ASSISTANCE :

2.1. Knowledge about Telecare :

Among the participants, only 14 (35.9%) had an idea about the concept of tele-assistance. (Figure 4)

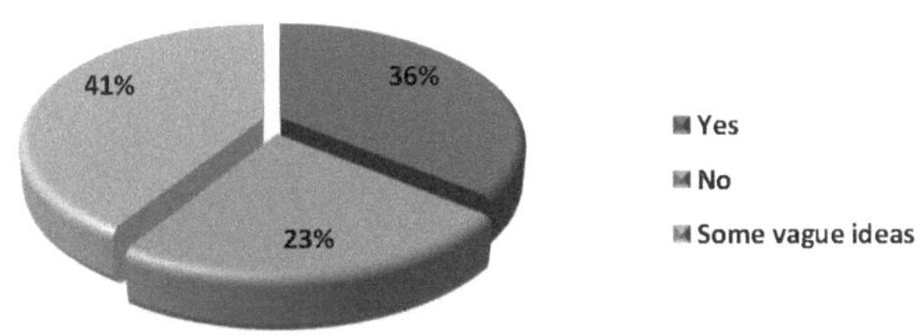

Figure 4: Distribution of the population according to their knowledge of telecare

2.2 Experience in Remote Assistance :

Most participants (57%) reported participating in videoconference surgery at least five times as a required physician or simple observer (see Figure 5).

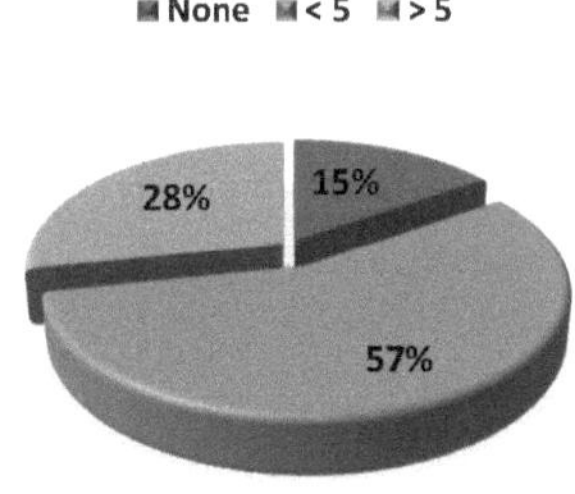

Figure 5: Distribution of the population according to their telecare experience

2.3. Benefits of remote assistance :

Thirty-one participants admitted to having gained new theoretical knowledge or improved surgical skills through their participation in surgical procedures via videoconferencing.

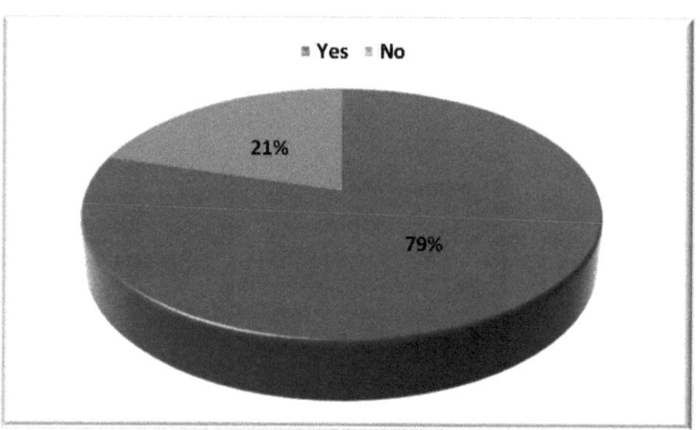

Figure 6: Distribution of the population according to their opinions on the educational benefits of telecare

2.4. Personal opinion on the use of tele-assistance in surgery :

Most participants (75.9%) saw tele-assistance as an excellent initiative. The different opinions are illustrated in Table 1.

Table I: Distribution of the population according to their opinion about videoconferencing

Opinion on videoconferencing	Number	Percentage
Excellent initiative	30	76,9%
Inconceivable	3	7,7%
Unethical	1	2,6%
Interesting	1	2,6%
Interesting in case of respect of ethical principles	1	2,6%
On a case by case basis	1	2,6%
No Idea	2	5%

3. ETHICAL ISSUES OF TELEHEALTH ASSISTANCE :

3.1 Telecare and respect for the patient's privacy and confidentiality:

Participants felt that video-conferencing tele-assistance in surgery was fully respectful of patient privacy in 38% of cases (Table 2).

In addition, 12 participants (30.8% of cases) felt that video-conferencing teleassistance in surgery respects patient confidentiality as shown in Table 2.

Table II: Distribution of the population according to their opinion regarding privacy and confidentiality during surgical teleassistance

Items	Staff	Percentage
Tele-assistance respects the patient's privacy		
Absolutely	15	38,5%
Not really	8	20,5%
Almost	16	41%
Not at all	0	0%
Tele-assistance respects the confidentiality of the patient's data.		
Absolutely	12	30,8%
Not really	10	25,6%
Almost	17	43,6%
Not at all	0	0%

3.2. Tele-assistance and information :

Of the participants, 30 (77% of cases) felt that it was mandatory to inform the patient about the procedure and the fact that it will be videotaped (see Figure 10).

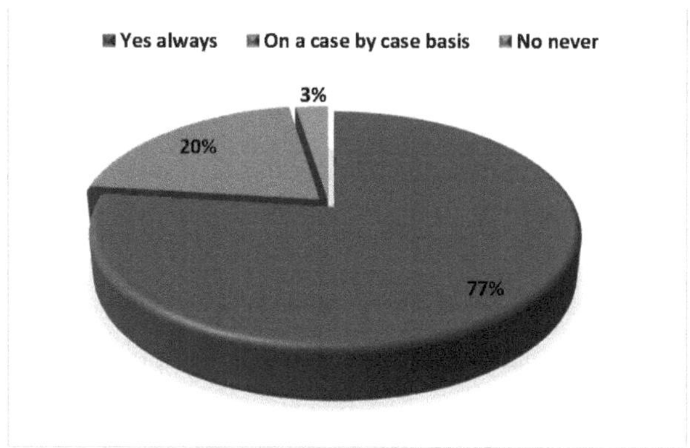

Figure 7: Distribution of the population by their opinion regarding patient information

3.3. Tele-assistance and consent :

Written patient consent is mandatory according to 31 participants (79% of cases). (Figure 11)

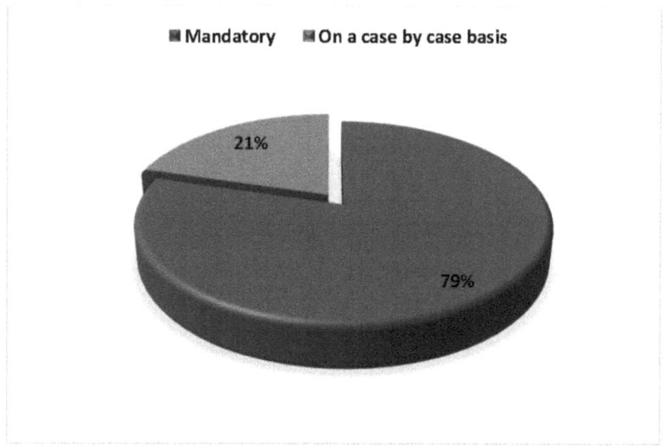

Figure 8: Distribution of Population by Opinion on the Need for Written Consent

3.4. Telecare and patient risk :

Of the participants, 23 or 59% thought that videoconferencing did not expose the patient to an additional risk of intraoperative incidents and complications compared to conventional surgery, as illustrated in the table below.

Table III: Distribution of the population according to their opinion regarding patient exposure to risks during surgery by tele-assistance

Tele-assistance: risk of additional incidents for the patient	Staff	Percentage
Absolutely	5	12,8%
Not really	8	20,5%
Almost	22	56,4%
Not at all	4	10,3%

3.5. Tele-assistance and medical liability :

Most of the participants (43.6%) thought that tele-assistance did not really expose the surgeon to any additional medico-legal risk and therefore to greater medical liability than with conventional surgery (Table IV).

Table IV: Distribution of the population according to their opinion regarding the engagement of medical liability in the case of videoconferencing

Tele-assistance: an additional source of medical responsibility	Staff	Percentage
Absolutely	9	23,1%
Not really	17	43,6%
Almost	9	23,1%
Not at all	4	10,3%

3.6. Tele-assistance and ethical standards :

More than half of the participants (61.5%) thought that videoconferencing surgery in its current form is virtually ethical (Table V).

Table V: Distribution of the population according to their opinion on the respect of ethical standards in the case of videoconferencing

Tele-assistance and respect for ethical standards	Staff	Percentage
Absolutely	5	12,8%
Not really	7	17,9%
Almost	24	61,5%
Not at all	3	7,7%

3.7. Opinion on the agreement to participate in a surgical operation by Teleassistance or its recommendation to a relative :

Most participants (n = 18) did not strongly agree with participating in a videoconference as a patient or recommending them to a relative (see Table 6).

Table VI: Distribution of the population according to their opinion about agreeing to participate in tele-assisted surgery or recommending it to a relative

Would you agree to be operated on (or would you recommend that a parent have the operation) by videoconference?	Staff	Percentage
Absolutely	12	30,2%
Not really	18	46,2%
Not at all	9	23,1%

Discussion

It emerges from our study that more than half of the participants (64.1% of the cases) have no knowledge or only vague ideas about telemedicine, more specifically tele-medical assistance, hence the interest of this work.

First of all, we believe it is wise to define the terms e-health and telemedicine and to detail the different fields of their application.

1. E-HEALTH, TELEMEDICINE: WHAT'S THE DIFFERENCE?

The terms telemedicine and telehealth or e-health are often confusing. For the World Health Organization (WHO), e-health is defined as "digital services for the well-being of the individual". It is also defined as "the use of tools for the production, transmission, management and sharing of digitized information for the benefit of both medical and medico-social practices".

Gunther Eysenbach [5] defines it as a set of communicating tools that strengthen the patient's ability to access quality care and to be an informed actor in the management of his or her health; it jointly improves caregivers' and patients' access to reliable information and changes the balance between caregivers and patients [6].

As for telemedicine, it was defined by the WHO in 1997 as "that part of medicine which uses the transmission by telecommunication of medical information (images, reports, recordings, etc.), with a view to remotely obtaining a diagnosis, specialized advice, continuous monitoring of a patient, a therapeutic decision".

Telehealth or e-health is therefore a broader term that includes telemedicine but also medico-social acts [3].

In 1996, Field et al. [7] highlighted the diversity of the fields of application of telemedicine by distinguishing between: clinical applications which concerned the management of a patient's medical situation, and non-clinical applications in the field of teaching, training, medical research and public health. In addition, five fields of application or disciplines of telemedicine can be distinguished:

1.1 Teleconsultation :

Teleconsultation is defined as "a medical act whose purpose is to enable a medical professional to give a remote consultation to a patient". This act is carried out in the presence of the patient who dialogues with the requesting physician and/or the required teleconsulting physician(s) [3]. The physician may have access to images of the patient (i.e. radiological and photographic images) via computer networks. Physician and patient can talk to each other by videophone. The patient's medical record in telehealth can be consulted remotely by the physician.

Example: remote consultation of an elderly person in a nursing home for elderly dependents (EHPAD) by the geriatrician of a hospital.

1.2 Tele-expertise :

Tele-expertise is defined as any diagnostic and/or therapeutic act that is performed outside the presence of the patient. The medical act of tele-expertise is described as an exchange between two or more physicians who together establish a diagnosis and/or therapy on the basis of clinical, radiological and/or biological data in a patient's medical record. It allows a medical professional (requesting physician) to request at a distance the opinion of one or more medical professionals (requested physician) because of their training or specific skills.

Example: requesting a neurosurgical opinion from an emergency room physician to a neurologist via videoconference to manage a stroke patient.

1.3. Remote medical monitoring :

Telemonitoring is a medical act that results from the transmission and interpretation by a physician of a clinical, radiological or biological indicator collected by the patient himself or by a health professional. The interpretation may lead to the decision to intervene with the patient. It is interpreted today by a physician, who may in the future delegate a course of action to another healthcare professional. This will be based on a written protocol for monitoring the said indicator which will have been validated by the attending physician or a physician required.

Example: remote monitoring of pregnant women through telemonitoring solutions that sends the patient's vitals to a health care facility while she remains at home.

1.4. Remote medical assistance :

Tele-assistance is conceived when a doctor remotely assists another doctor performing a medical or surgical procedure. The physician may also assist another health professional who is performing a medical or imaging procedure, or even, in the case of an emergency, remotely assist a first-aid worker or any person providing assistance to a person in danger while waiting for a physician to arrive. Tele-assistance procedures are already well established in several specialties. Surgery is more and more remotely controlled thanks to robotics, especially in visceral cancer microsurgery. Procedures currently performed by laparoscopy can be improved by remote assistance. Remote assistance also concerns procedures performed by a non-physician assisted by a physician. The fibrinolysis of a patient with a stroke before transfer to a Neurovascular Unit is a very concrete case. It is associated with a teleconsultation situation for the neurologist in relation to the suspected stroke.

1.5. Remote control :

It is the medical response provided within the framework of the medical regulation of emergencies or the permanence of care.

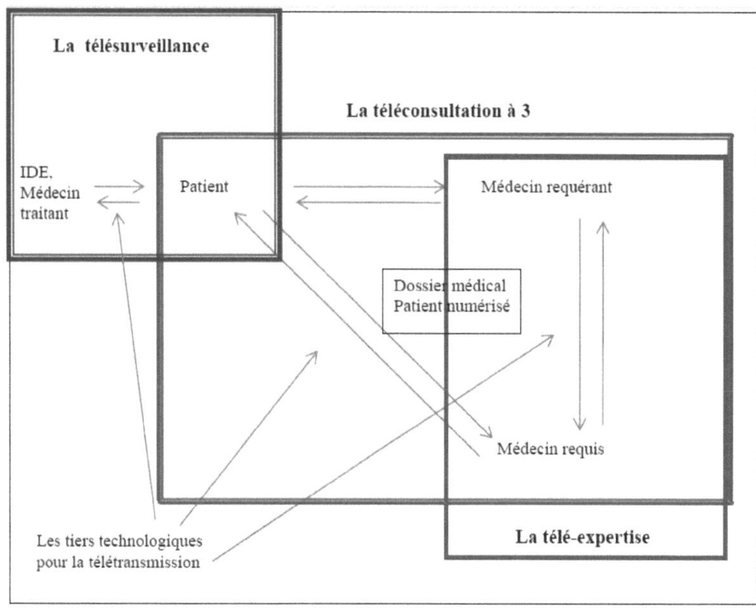

Figure 9: Summary of the obligations that unite the different actors involved in the three main telemedicine medical acts (brown frame for telemonitoring, red frame for teleconsultation, green frame for tele-expertise). [3]

2. BENEFITS OF TELEMEDICINE :

Telemedicine seems to make up for the various shortcomings of the health system. It enables the optimization of the healthcare system by acting on its different actors.

2.1. Patients :

Telemedicine allows for more reliable and coordinated care, a reduction in the number of examinations, a reduction in the number of unjustified emergency room visits, easier home care for people suffering from chronic pathologies and continuity of care.

It offers the opportunity for better access to care in areas of low medical density. Finally, all these advantages contribute to improving the doctor-patient relationship [8].

2.2. Health care professionals and institutions :

For healthcare professionals, telemedicine offers a better use of purely medical time and invaluable decision and diagnostic support tools. It also enables the continuing education of physicians through access to validated medical knowledge resources and enriches physicians' professional and personal experience through the possibility of teamwork and the exchange of information and experience. It contributes to the decompartmentalization between city medicine, hospitals and the medico-social sector in a care pathway logic.

3. REGULATORY FRAMEWORK OF TELEMEDICINE IN TUNISIA AND IN THE WORLD :

In Tunisia, and in many other countries, laws are in place to protect citizens' health data and respect their confidentiality.

3.1 Regulatory framework of e-health in Tunisia :

3.1.1. Legal framework :

In Tunisia, telemedicine is essentially governed by the order of the Minister of Public Health of 15 May 1996, establishing and organizing the technical committee of telemedicine [9]. Indeed, this committee is responsible for giving its opinion on any telemedicine project in the structures under the authority of the Ministry of Public Health, particularly in the field of :
- Development of the telemedicine strategy and programs of the Ministry of Public Health,
- To determine the measures necessary for the implementation, execution and evaluation of the programs established in the field of telemedicine.
On the other handlaw n° 2018-43 of July 11, 2018, supplementing the law n° 91-21 of March 13, 1991, relating to the exercise and organization of the profession of physician and dentist [10] stipulates in its article 23 bis that the physician or dentist can practice his profession within the framework of telemedicine. The modification of article 23 of

law n°91-21 had introduced telemedicine as a sixth type of authorized medical act for medical professionals. This law also defined telemedicine as *"the remote medical practice using information and communication technologies to bring together, among themselves or with a patient, doctors or dentists and other health professionals, which necessarily includes a physician, and where appropriate, other treating health professionals, in particular to establish a diagnosis of a disease, to collect a medical opinion, to monitor or follow up a patient's condition, or other medical services and acts. "»* [10]

Given the particular context of the Covid-19 pandemic and the justified and important need of the population to have an alternative to ensure remote medical care, the National Council of the Medical Order of Tunisia (CNOM) has issued an opinion on telemedicine. In its first press release, dated March 15, 2020, entitled "Covid19: recommendations to the medical profession", the CNOM has authorized the practice of telemedicine. The CNOM thus specifies that the physician may use remote consultation, telecommunication, video-conferencing and remote prescription renewal for chronic pathologies [11]. These authorizations have been given to reduce congestion in the healthcare circuit and facilitate medical practice. This authorization is exceptional and limited in time (until the end of the pandemic). The CNOM recalled in a second press release dated April 18, 2020 that the order had a single platform with the Ministry of Health designated, within the framework of a partnership, through which teleconsultations will be authorized [12]. This platform offers free access to avoid conflict of interest and commits to transfer all data recorded to the Ministry of Health at the end of the pandemic and to keep no copies [12].

3.1.2. Ethical framework :

In July 2017, the Conseil National de l'Ordre des Médecins (CNOM) published a charter setting out the main ethical rules for the use of digital media by physicians [13]. 13] In this charter, the CNOM authorizes and encourages the use of digital media in compliance with the ethical rules common to the practice of medicine. Its objective is to provide a framework for the digitalization of medical practice and the use of online digital media. However, Chapter IV of this charter imposes the need to respect the patient-patient relationship. Indeed, a medical consultation necessarily requires an examination of the patient. Any information or advice given online does not constitute a medical consultation. However, as stated in article 19 of this charter [13], it is deontologically acceptable for a physician to use information and communication technology to answer a question asked by the patient following a consultation.

However, and in the absence of implementing legislation, telemedicine legislation does not provide a sufficient legal basis. It exposes its beneficiaries to specific medico-legal issues and risks that are often additional to the risks inherent in conventional medical practice.

3.2 Regulatory framework of telemedicine in the world :

In France, telemedicine was defined for the first time in article 32 of law n° 2004-810 of August 13, 2004 [14] as a remote medical act: *"telemedicine makes it possible, among other things, to perform medical acts in strict compliance with the rules of deontology but at a distance, under the control and responsibility of a doctor in contact with the patient by means of communication appropriate to the medical act"*. Then, the law of July 21, 2009, known as the HPST law [15] dedicated a legal framework to the practice of telemedicine in its article 78. Article L. 6316-1. defines telemedicine as *"a form of remote medical practice using information and communication technologies. It brings one or more healthcare professionals into contact with one another or with a patient, including necessarily a medical professional and, where appropriate, other professionals providing care to the patient. »*

It stipulates that *"It enables a diagnosis to be established, a preventive or post-treatment follow-up for a patient at risk to be carried out, a specialist opinion to be sought, a therapeutic decision to be prepared, products to be prescribed, services or procedures to be prescribed or performed, or the condition of patients to be monitored".*

Decree no. 2010-1229 of October 19, 2010 [16] defines telemedicine acts and the conditions for their implementation.

Similarly, Canada has federal legislation on the protection of online privacy, personal information and electronic documents [17].

Malaysia is one of the few developing countries with e-health legislation. Malaysia's Telemedicine Act 564 of 1997 regulates and controls the practice of telemedicine and all related issues [18].

The World Medical Association has a telemedicine policy that addresses the international practice of telemedicine [19]. The policies developed by this group over several years reflect the tension between ideal goals and technical limitations, as well as the complexity and evolution of e-health policies.

4. REGULATORY ISSUES IN TELEMEDICINE :

The practice of telemedicine in our country as in the world is not devoid of medico-legal risks. These problems may be related to the very organization of telemedicine, to the technological tools used in the various acts of telemedicine, or to the particularity of telemedicine, which is not necessarily conceived in a singular colloquium in its classical sense [20].

4.1. Telemedicine and the right of access to care :

The right to health care is a fundamental right for all citizens regardless of their social category. The practice of telemedicine, while challenging the traditional perception of the doctor-patient relationship, is also accompanied by a "duty of care" on the part of the doctor during a remote consultation between doctor and patient as in any other traditional medical consultation.

The main objective of the enactment of Law 2018-43 [21] was to facilitate access to quality health care on an equal basis for all Tunisian citizens regardless of their region. It provided that telemedicine could connect doctors to each other, the patient to a doctor or to a health professional(s), including necessarily at least one doctor, in order to diagnose a disease, obtain a medical opinion, ensure the monitoring or follow-up of a patient or other medical services and procedures [21]. 21] Thus, it appears that telemedicine will improve the quality of care provided to patients by facilitating consultation for patients who cannot travel or for obtaining expert advice. Moreover, 75.9% of the surgeons who participated in the survey thought that tele-assistance, one of the fields of application of telemedicine, was an excellent initiative. Moreover, 59% of them thought that it does not expose the patient to an additional risk of intra-operative incidents and complications compared to conventional surgery.

However, the lack of direct physical contact with the patient can sometimes affect the quality of care provided in terms of collecting signs and data from the physical examination. Therefore, it is essential that the physician supervise the protocols used. In addition, the setting up of conferences and the analysis of medical files is necessary in all health care institutions and in all circumstances. In addition, the physician should be able to immediately contact non-physician providers, technicians and patients. And with each telemedicine act, he or she should assess whether the situation requires direct contact with the patient in order to ensure quality of care.

4.2 Telemedicine and medical confidentiality :

According to our survey, only 38% of surgeons think that the tele-assistance act respects the patient's privacy. Similarly, 30.8% of them think that this act respects the confidentiality of the patient's data. Indeed, in Tunisia as in several other countries, issues relating to confidentiality and protection of personal data are a legal concern and they can engage medical liability. Article 254 of the Tunisian Penal Code (CPT) [22] and Articles 8 and 9 of the Code of Medical Ethics (CDM) [23] impose an obligation on physicians to protect the confidentiality of information to which they have had access during the practice of their profession. Moreover, physicians practicing in public health institutions also have an obligation of confidentiality under article 7 of Law No. 83-112 of December 12, 1983 [24]. In the field of telemedicine, law n° 2018-43 [21] has specified that telemedicine should only be practiced using computer systems and secure means of communication that guarantee the protection, security and authenticity of the documents, personal data and health-related data being exchanged. On the other hand, to better promote the protection of personal data in Tunisia, Article 1 of Organic Law No. 63 of July 27, 2004 on the protection of personal data stipulates that "*All persons have the right to the protection of personal data relating to their private life as one of the fundamental rights guaranteed by the Constitution and may only be processed in the context of transparency, fairness, and respect for human dignity and in accordance with the provisions of this law.* This protection applies to both digital and paper data. According to this law, the transfer or sharing of data can only take place after obtaining the patient's consent and authorization from the National Data Protection Authority (INDPP)[25]. 25] In addition, a draft organic law No. 25/2018 [26] has been proposed. It stipulates in Article 70 that "*Connected objects imported or locally manufactured and intended for marketing are subject to certification and compliance with the standards adopted for the protection of personal data in accordance with the legislation in force.* "Article 71 states that "*The Authority shall establish the conditions of protection by decision after consultation with the structures responsible for control and regulation in the field of electronic telecommunications.* ». In addition, the ratification of Convention 108 of the Council of Europe in May 2017 has enabled, in accordance with Article 20 of the Tunisian Constitution, to give it greater force than national law. Thus, several provisions of the law were amended or repealed by the mere fact of the entry into force of the said convention: Articles 53 and 54, which allowed public structures to benefit from a derogatory regime, or Article 16, which did the same for employers. According to the INDPP, Tunisia is the 51st member of Convention 108 of the Council of Europe. It is one of the first countries outside the European Union to apply the new law on the protection of personal data.

Worldwide, and more specifically in Europe, a new regulation on the protection of individuals with regard to the processing of personal data was adopted on April 27, 2016 and applied as of May 25, 2018 [27]. 27] This directive has brought greater harmonization at the European level. It clearly defined the rights and responsibilities of the entities in charge of data processing while adapting to current technological requirements.

In the United States, personal health data is governed by the Health Insurance Portability and Accountability Act (HIPPA). 28] HIPPA provides security rules for any health care provider who processes health information in electronic format. According to the rules defined by HIPAA, an entity (health care provider, health service provider, etc.) is responsible for the security of patient data. This implies that an application or service that collects, processes, and stores patient data must ensure the confidentiality and integrity of the data and impose access restrictions.

However, even with this legal panel, confidentiality and protection of patient data remains a concern for all telemedicine acts. As a result, it is important that the technologies and equipment used in telemedicine are not used by unauthorized persons or placed in conditions or locations that allow access by unauthorized persons. Therefore, it is the physician's responsibility to assess whether the technologies used to communicate with his or her patient in the context of telemedicine or with a third party are capable of maintaining professional secrecy [19]. 19] Similarly, the physician had to inform those assisting him or her, in particular the personnel in charge of the technical aspect and their obligation of medical secrecy. A patient's waiver of confidentiality or authorization to exchange information electronically does not relieve the physician of his or her duty to ensure, as far as possible, that professional secrecy is respected. On the other hand, exchanges between the patient and his or her treating physician as well as between the various health professionals involved in patient management must be secure in order to remain confidential. This implies the use of a business card or personal identifier that formally identifies the persons accessing the technology in question and their various actions, which should be traceable afterwards.

4.3. The computerized medical record (DMI) :

In any medical act, the keeping of medical records and documentation is mandatory in Tunisia regardless of the mode and place of practice [29].

This is obviously the case for the practice of telemedicine. In addition to the data of the clinical examination and the results of the complementary examinations, it is preferable that videoconferences are also recorded in the DMI. Indeed, the medical record is the main source of information for the evaluation of medical practices. In addition, it represents the cornerstone of communication between health care professionals.

The maintenance of computerized medical records raises the issue of confidentiality and data security [30]. 30] As a result, some countries such as Canada have established the characteristics of the electronic record [31]. 31] Indeed, the record must be protected by an access code specific to each user while allowing for the permanent availability of data and systems and protecting the integrity of the data to ensure data confidentiality. In addition, it must allow the identification of all users and the logging of accesses, guarantee the inalterability of transactions, and allow the transfer of data to another platform in a universal format [31]. On the other hand, the DMI also poses the problem of archiving [32]. Indeed, it is recommended that for each file there is in addition to the standard copy, a second copy called backup copy. In addition, it would also be necessary to guarantee the existence and security of back-up copies while preventing that, when transporting their media, they cannot be read, copied, modified, erased or deleted. If necessary, the responsibility of the health care institution, the physician and also the provider of the IT service could be engaged.

4.4. Telemedicine, information and consent :

Most of the surgeons who participated in the survey (77% of the cases) thought that informing the patient of the modalities and procedures in case of tele-assistance and video recording of the procedure is mandatory. In addition, 79% thought that consent must be obtained in writing. Indeed, in Tunisia, information and consent constitute a moral, ethical and legal obligation. They are governed by several legislative texts. These include the Patients' Charter "MSP circular n°36 of May 19, 2009" [13], decree n°81-1634 of November 30, 1981 [29], concerning the general internal regulations of hospitals and case law (Tunis Court of Appeals rulings 48788 of April 29, 1998 and n°95747 of June 4, 2003, Criminal Cassation Court rulings n°36624 of June 25, 2003 and n°20241 of March 13, 2013). On the other hand, the Code of Medical Ethics (CDM) implicitly insinuates the obligation to inform the patient and to obtain his consent before any action is taken [23].

In the field of telemedicine, Law No. 2018-43 insisted on the need for information and consent in all areas of telemedicine application. It stipulates that the doctor or dentist in charge must not perform any act in the context of telemedicine unless he has informed the patient and, where appropriate, his legal guardian. In such cases, the nature of the information goes beyond the known field of conventional medicine and relates to the patient's state of health and the care proposed. The information must also cover data relating to the technologies to be used, the rate of access to these technologies, their accessibility and ease of use. On the other hand, the physician must also inform the patient of his or her share of the work in the event of tele-monitoring, the need to be assisted by others, and the need to seek advice from colleagues in the context of tele-expertise or tele-assistance. In addition, this law stresses the importance of collecting informed consent by any means that leaves a written or electronic record, except for the exceptions cited in the Tunisian medical code of ethics such as a vital emergency or in the event that it proves impossible to obtain consent.

4.5. Telemedicine and medical liability :

The act of telemedicine constitutes a medical act in its own right, in terms of its indication and quality. It is not a degraded form of it. As a result, the physician may be held liable in case of non-compliance with legal and ethical standards.

4.5.1. Medical responsibility in teleconsultation :

As far as teleconsultation is concerned, it must be of at least equivalent, if not superior, quality to the quality of traditional medical acts. Indeed, telemedicine makes the possibilities of access to care faster and wider and thus improves the means available to the patient's doctor to practice his art. Of course, the physician is bound by an obligation of means and not of results. However, the physician must judge the level of care provided via telehealth to be correct and at least equivalent to any other type of care that may be provided to the patient, taking into account the context, location, time and relative availability of conventional care. If the level of care is not deemed appropriate via tele-consultation, the physician should inform the patient and suggest an alternative mode of care. If a decision is made to use telemedicine, it is necessary to ensure that the users (patients and health professionals) are able to use the necessary telecommunication system. The physician should seek to ensure that the patient has understood the advice and treatment suggestions given and take steps where possible to promote continuity of care.

In addition, it is necessary for the physician to clearly and explicitly inform the patient, in the presence of other health care providers involved, who is responsible for the follow-up and ongoing treatment.

A physician whose advice is sought through telemedicine must keep a detailed record of the advice he or she gives and the information received and on which the advice was based in order to ensure traceability.

4.5.2. Medical responsibility in tele-expertise :

This is a new field of medical responsibility. The physician may in certain cases propose the consultation of a colleague as soon as the circumstances require it or when he considers that his capacities are exceeded.

In this mode of telemedicine practice, the responsibility involved may be that of the requesting physician, who will be the one who makes the final decision on diagnostic or therapeutic matters. The latter is also responsible for the information collected and transmitted [33]. 33] It may be the responsibility of the requested physician if it turns out that he or she has given an opinion outside his or her field of expertise, if he or she has committed a fault on his or her part, or if he or she has committed a fault in relation to missing or inadequate elements or a technical problem without having mentioned it to the requesting physician. Finally, liability may be joint and several and shared if it appears that the fault was committed at both levels [33,34]. In all cases, both medical professionals should strive to act with probity and diligence. They should clarify situations that may interfere with their decision or even refrain from giving an opinion or making a decision when necessary [33]. In all cases, the requesting physician must inform the patient before sharing data with anyone, respect the patient's wishes and obtain the patient's consent before sharing information about the patient. In addition, the report of a tele-expertise procedure must include the name and signature of the expert consulted or physician required. Case law will certainly adjust the responsibilities involved more clearly as practices evolve.

4.5.3. Medical liability in the field of telemonitoring :

One of the main applications of telemonitoring is in the monitoring of chronic diseases. The first step in this practice is the collection of the indicator, an act carried out by the patient or by an informed professional. The latter is responsible for carrying out this mission. Indeed, although the tools used in the transmission of monitoring indicators are subject to a compliance and safety requirement, in the event of a malfunction, the professional must declare the incident in order to discharge himself of responsibility. In the second stage of remote monitoring, the physician interprets the indicator. This is an intellectual medical act. The attending physician is obliged to use reliable and certified equipment [33,35]. 33,35] However, he or she may incur liability.

4.5.4. Medical responsibility in telecare :

In 43.6% of the cases, the participants in our survey thought that operating with the help of videoconferencing assistance does not really expose the surgeon to any additional medico-legal risk. In fact, the liability regime for teleassistance is the same as for procedures performed within the framework of teleconsultation or teleexpertise. In cases where one doctor assists another doctor via telemedicine, the responsibilities for the diagnostic or therapeutic act are often shared.

4.5.5. Medical liability in the field of teleregulation :

Medical answers provided to callers by telephone are now considered to be simple medical advice. In the future, medical regulation could evolve towards teleconsultation through videoconferencing. The legal responsibility would fall to the establishment hosting the medical regulation center for the permanence of care.

5. TELEMEDICINE AND ETHICAL ISSUES :

More than half of the participants (61.5%) thought that tele-assistance by videoconference in its current form meets ethical standards. In this work, we propose to discuss the ethical issues not only of telecare but of all the fields of application of telemedicine. To do so, our ethical approach is mainly based on the discussion of the four ethical principles of Beauchamp and Childress [36]: beneficence, autonomy, non-maleficence and justice. These elements are conceived both as tools for solving human problems and as guidelines for integrating the ethical dimension into practices. The quality of the capture, storage and use of medical data in health care institutions, on the one hand, and the different fields of application of telemedicine, on the other hand, must be the subject of an explicit requirement instituted in an ethical charter [37]. 37] In this context, this ethical prism makes it possible to better apprehend and understand the paradox that exists between the promotion of the health of the individual through the application of new technologies and the harmful repercussions that they may induce.

5.1. Charity :

Beneficence is a fundamental principle of medical ethics. This principle of beneficence is understood as "the moral obligation to act for the good of others. Telemedicine aims to improve the patient's quality of life first and foremost by promoting easier access to care. From now on, patients are no longer obliged to travel to health institutions to monitor their chronic pathologies through telemonitoring. In 2019, a major study conducted by French researchers analyzed the perception and opinion of 1,200 patients with various chronic conditions about the use of artificial intelligence and portable biometric monitoring devices: 47% thought they were a great step forward, while 11% saw them as a danger [38]. Remote monitoring does not only allow remote monitoring of patients' vital signs, but through this technology, healthcare professionals also accompany their patients in their daily lives and advise them on new lifestyle habits that are considered "healthier". On the other hand, the appropriate dissemination of medical knowledge to the user of the computer system, whether healthcare professionals or patients, constitutes a justification and legitimacy of action. Patients can learn more about their pathology and the right behaviors. Their culture is enriched. Thus, medical communication, and therefore the management of care, becomes more effective. A report published in 2001 by the US Institute of Medicine (US Institute of Medicine) established a particular link between information technology, improved healthcare delivery and improved communication with patients and clinicians. The ability of patients to manage their own care would be enhanced if they had more information about their health [39]. Moreover, in geographical areas that are difficult to access, the patient has the right to be consulted by the appropriate experts through teleconsultation and can even be operated on. A powerful illustration of the impact of telemedicine on improving the quality of care occurred after Hurricane Katrina in the United States. In the four days following the hurricane, the Veterans Health Administration was able to transfer the records of 50,000 patients from the flooded hospital and clinics in New Orleans, Louisiana to Houston, Texas [40]. The National Health Information Technology Coordinator worked with pharmacies to create a drug database for 800,000 people in the storm-affected area. This connectivity supported continuity of care and access to care. In addition, the computerization of medical records would bring enormous time savings and easier access. In a study in the United Kingdom, patients felt that IMRs could help ensure continuity of care, particularly in emergency situations [41].

However, this benevolent intention is not devoid of ethical issues. One may question the legitimacy of health professionals to determine, for a third person, living conditions and a particular way of life because of his or her illness. Indeed, who can be better placed than the patient to evaluate the quality of life to which he or she aspires according to his or her life project, values and beliefs? And on what basis can the intervention of caregivers in the area of patient privacy be justified? Doesn't the computerization of patients' personal data and the fact of being able to share them constitute an infringement of the patient's privacy? Finally, what guarantees do we have concerning the security of this data and the preservation of medical secrecy?

5.2. Autonomy :

The emergence of telemedicine was initially influenced by the desire to promote patient autonomy. According to Beauchamp and Childress, autonomy is the ability to act on one's own by giving oneself one's own rules of conduct, one's own law. Consequently, the autonomous individual "acts freely in accordance with a project that he himself has chosen" [36]. It is also the right to self-determination. The purpose of this principle is to involve the patient in the decision-making process. The emergence of new medical practices in the context of telemedicine is reconsidering the notion of care, by considering it in a more global way by integrating all the acts whose purpose is the well-being of the sick person. Indeed, telemedicine integrates the daily life of the patient with his or her behavior, lifestyle habits and values. The patient's life project and lifestyle are necessarily taken into account by the caregivers in order to best personalize the care and, above all, to precisely determine the nature of their action. On the other hand, the principle of autonomy presupposes that the patient makes a conscious decision to adhere to his or her care. Informed consent is a typical example of autonomy. Informed consent is evidence of conscious and informed decision making. In addition, autonomy also includes the patient's right to access and correct his or her record and to authorize others who may have access to it [42].

However, this principle of autonomy is not always respected. Indeed, it is necessary to question the paradox existing between the will to make the patient more autonomous and the need to change his or her life habits. Moreover, it is essential to underline that telemedicine is increasingly intervening in the private life and intimacy of the patient. This approach is not without problems from an ethical point of view and may undermine respect for the patient's autonomy. On the other hand, when exposed to the disease, the individual becomes more fragile and vulnerable. Making decisions about their health status can be difficult and in some cases impossible. Health care personnel must ensure that they provide the necessary information regarding the therapeutic modalities and the consequences of different choices. They should support the patient in making decisions and respect the patient's choices. In addition, the computerization of health data introduces other considerations related to autonomy. One of these considerations is the extent to which patients want their data to be shared in databases or integrated into a national health database. Indeed, in a study conducted in the UK, 16% of participants identified health problems that they did not wish to share [43]. Another study in the United Kingdom showed that 50% of the respondents were concerned that their records would be linked outside their doctor's office [44]. Indeed, patients provide data to health care staff for specific reasons. Combining these data to create new information about these same patients without their knowledge or permission violates the principle of autonomy.

5.3. Justice :

This principle is closely related to the notions of equality and equity. Telemedicine can be an extraordinary opportunity for greater equality of opportunity to access care in all countries of the world. It has shown in several countries a return of general practitioners to areas deserted by them because they can organize telemedicine assistance from remote health care centers. It also allows for a globalization of access to specialists and a common work in teams of doctors at the service of the patient.

There are stimulating experiences. Remote rural areas deserted by physicians have shown the usefulness of direct interactions between patients and physicians via telemedicine. Remote care exists for many specialties. In developing countries and Eastern Europe, access to specialized centers in areas not readily available at home, such as teleradiology, can be an important step forward. In the event of a major disaster, tsunami, nuclear contamination, earthquakes, doctors can no longer move around, they have to stay on site and the presence of previously experienced robots makes it possible to treat patients not only for diagnosis but also for treatment, including surgery. In all countries remote monitoring allows to follow chronic diseases. This exists in Belgium for kidney failure, in Holland for diabetes. The miniaturization of the sensors allows a better telemonitoring and tele-nursing. The services considered as still experimental but which exist, are remote surgery in ophthalmology as well as in digestive surgery and neurosurgery. Among the demonstrations of the effectiveness and globalization of telemedicine we mention in Belgium, teleradiology in Mechelen and teledialysis in France and Germany, telemonitoring in Dijon and Heidelberg, in the United Kingdom a national telehealth program, in the United States of America, teleHealth neuro-cardio-imaging self-management with, as a pioneer, the Mayo Clinic in Rochester and the Kaiser Permanente Foundation in California and Canada, laparoscopic telerobotics for abdominal surgery in Ontario. Vast countries such as Australia have enabled the development of a national broadband network with synchronous teleconsultations and asynchronous delayed dispatch recordings. Countries requesting and in the process of international development are in North Africa and the Middle East, Morocco and Algeria and Egypt.

In addition, telemedicine and, on a larger scale, telehealth help to identify socio-economic and racial discrimination in the delivery of health services [45]. Therefore, once identified, these inequalities could be addressed through health policies. However, justice may also be violated through the distribution of electronic resources and the inequitable public disclosure of personal health information of certain disadvantaged groups. Some authors have referred to the "digital divide" between those who have computers and Internet access and those who do not [46]. 46] People with computers and Internet access will be able to use online health information resources [47]. Economic status is not the only disincentive to access information and communication technologies. Age is also a factor. A national survey in the United States found that 69% of people aged 65 and over had never been online [48]. 48] In addition, the percentage of people aged 75 and over was 82%. These people often have chronic illnesses and could make the most of online health information and online communication with health care workers [49].

Another group of researchers discovered another source of imbalance related to health ministry websites. U.S. state governments have used websites to provide health information to their citizens. States also allow their citizens to access information such as quality data on health providers and to request services such as eligibility criteria, forms, and interpreters through these websites [47]. The researchers found that the websites did not provide equitable access in terms of readability for people with disabilities, translations for non-English-speaking readers, and geographic distribution of the web [47]. 47] Other researchers have found that people with lower incomes, lower education, or African-Americans have less access to the Internet [50]. 50] These individuals will then be underserved by public health services.

5.4. Non-maleficence :

This principle aims to avoid harm to the person for whom one is responsible, to spare him or her from harm or suffering. Its purpose therefore implies doing good or refraining from doing harm. The contribution of computerization to the field of health could be in contradiction with the ethical principle of non-maleficence. Indeed, although telemedicine allows much greater speed and ease of access to care with faster or more appropriate treatment, it may also threaten the confidentiality of patients' personal or health-related information [51]. In hospital IT, the risks and abuses that may have occurred were mainly linked to the excessive number of managers of all kinds and their lack of competence in the field of IT. Among the major risks is also the transmission of information via the Internet, in particular the disclosure of personal data such as the social security number, which could be used by mutual health insurance companies to select their own clients based on their medical history. Because of this, France has argued that personal health information should "only be consulted by authorized persons, for well-defined purposes, taking into account the interests of the patient" [51]. 51] In addition, health care personnel are required to maintain the confidentiality and security of health information, including data contained in computerized medical records. In a study conducted in the United Kingdom, 50% of patients were concerned about the security of their electronic records [44]. 44] These participants had good reason to be concerned. Unfortunately, the popular press in the United States is replete with violations of this obligation [52,53]. In the United States, the Privacy Rights Clearinghouse [54] monitors security breaches, particularly those involving the national identifier, the Social Security Number. Between January and November 2006, the organization recorded more than 27 health data security breaches involving more than 900,000 individuals.

Non-maleficence can also be broken when research and epidemiological studies are published. For example, the publication of detailed maps of diseases and health conditions may compromise confidentiality [55]. Current Geographic Information System (GIS) software capabilities are so accurate that single-family home addresses can be identified with 79% and 100% accuracy within 14 meters [55]. The lack of privacy protection for health data is the result of multiple situations. Health data are exposed when security measures are inadequate. Individuals become identifiable in presentation formats. Some countries advocate limited access to personal health data according to the profile and nature of the user to improve the security, confidentiality and protection of such data. However, this selective arrangement of personal health data has a negative impact on the principle of Justice, because the medical information transmitted is not the same depending on the user of the database. In a way, this reflects a discrimination of individuals and a hierarchy of medical data leading to an asymmetry of medical knowledge, and therefore calls into question the transparency of medical information. In order to guarantee this non-maleficence, it will be necessary to respect the legislative regulation of medical data, to respect the rules of storage, hosting and dissemination of personal data. In addition, care must be taken to ensure the reliability of the collection of medical data and its permanence, as well as the technical relevance and human merits of the tool. On the other hand, telemedicine can also be harmful to patients because it exposes them to the risk of a dehumanization of the caregiver/patient relationship. Many people question the quality of the care relationship in the context of remote care. How can we be sure that we are not satisfied with the patient's clinical elements alone? And is it possible to consider factors as sensitive and personal as the patient's emotions or feelings through a non-presential interview with the caregiver?

Conclusion

The emergence of telemedicine is undoubtedly a fundamental advance in the practice of medicine. It represents a powerful leverage arm allowing the restructuring of the Tunisian health system and constitutes a non-negligible solution in terms of responses to various public health problems such as medical desertification. Moreover, telemedicine improves the quality of life of patients by limiting their travel and allowing them to consult their doctor remotely, to be monitored more regularly through a remote monitoring device or to benefit from the opinion of one or more experts via tele-expertise.

However, the practice of telemedicine is not yet well developed in Tunisia. This can be explained to some extent by the legal vagueness that surrounds it and the regulatory issues it may represent. Indeed, the computerization of medical records containing patient information and the integration of new non health professional actors such as technological third parties or access providers, is not without problems in terms of organization of care and respect for patient rights, especially with regard to privacy and medical confidentiality. Moreover, the lack of hindsight and the lack of knowledge of caregivers regarding the issue of their legal responsibility in the practice of telemedicine, raise fears of mistrust and reluctance of health professionals to practice these new medical practices. However, it is true that, to date, there is no specific regime for the legal liability of health professionals practicing telemedicine. Further clarification is needed in this regard. An evolution of Tunisian law is desirable in view of the particularities of these new medical practices and more particularly in view of the provisions relating to professional secrecy and confidentiality of patient health data. On the other hand, telemedicine also raises important ethical questions. It is undeniable that it provides healthcare professionals with numerous innovative care tools aimed at making patients more autonomous in their care. Moreover, the various telemedicine acts aim to respond as well as possible to the different demands of patients, based mainly on improving their quality of life and ensuring equity of care for all individuals. However, these fundamental ethical principles are sometimes threatened. Concerns about the protection of privacy, confidentiality and even intimacy arise, which can harm the beneficiaries of telemedicine services and call into question the respect of ethical standards.

In conclusion, dialogue with the patient must be privileged. Clear and fair information to the patient must not be lacking. Respect for confidentiality and privacy is a legal, ethical and deontological obligation that must always be respected. The physician providing telehealth care must ensure compliance with legislation and professional guidelines on telemedicine. In addition to being competent in the relevant field of practice, the physician should be able to communicate well, understand the purpose of the service provided via telemedicine, understand the protocols and procedures of telemedicine, and be aware of the limitations of the technology used. For ignoring or neglecting these issues exposes to the risk of harming patients and the commitment of the responsibility of healthcare professionals.

References

1. Organisation Mondiale de la Santé. A health telematics policy in support of WHO's Health-for-all strategy for global health development : report of the WHO Group Consultation on Health Telematics [Internet]. Geneva: OMS; 1998 [cité 25 nov 2020] p. 39. Report No.: WHO/DGO/98.1. Disponible sur: https://apps.who.int

2. Dupagne D. E-santé. Communications. 2011;88(1):57.

3. Simon P, Acker D. The place of telemedicine in the organization of care. Paris: Department of Health and Sports; 2008.

4. Chopard J-L, Hubert N, Moulin T, Medeiros de Bustos E. Legal, deontological and ethical issues applied to telemedicine. A few insights about telestroke. Eur Res Telemed Rech Eur En Télémédecine. juin 2012;1(2):61-5.

5. Eysenbach G. What is e-health? J Med Internet Res. June 18, 2001;3(2):e20.

6. WHO Global Observatory for eHealth, World Health Organization. MHealth: new horizons for health through mobile technologies. [Internet]. Geneva: World Health Organization; 2011 [cité 25 nov 2020]. Disponible sur: http://www.who.int/goe/publications/goe_mhealth_web.pdf

7. Field MJ. Telemedicine: A Guide to Assessing Telecommunications for Health Care [Internet]. Washington, D.C.: National Academies Press; 1996 [cité 25 nov 2020]. Disponible sur: http://www.nap.edu/catalog/5296

8. Schleyer TKL, Spallek H, Bartling WC, Corby P. The technologically well-equipped dental office. J Am Dent Assoc. janv 2003;134(1):30-41.

9. Official Printing Office of the Republic of Tunisia. Order of the Minister of Public Health of May 15, 1996, on the creation and organization of the technical committee of telemedicine. Official Journal of the Tunisian Republic May 24, 1996 p. 1040-5.

10. Official Printing Office of the Republic of Tunisia. Law n° 91-21 of March 13, 1991, relating to the exercise and organization of the profession of physician and dentist. Official Journal of the Tunisian Republic March 15, 1991 p. 408-11.

11- National Council of the Medical Order of Tunisia. Communiqué of the National Council of the Medical Order. Covid19 : recommendations to the medical profession. Internet]. March 15, 2020. Available at: http://www.ordre-medecins.org.tn/fr/

12. National Council of the Tunisian Medical Association. Communiqué of the National Council of the Medical Order. About Telemedicine. Internet]. Apr 18, 2020. Available at: http://www.ordre-medecins.org.tn/fr/

13. Patients' Charter in Tunisia. Ministry of Health Tunisia [Internet]. Available at: http://www.santetunisie.rns.tn/

14. DELPRAT L. Law No. 2004-810 of August 13, 2004 on health insurance reform, issues and prospects. Rev DROIT SANTE. 2005;(6):270-81.

15. Law No. 2009-879 of July 21, 2009, on hospital reform and relating to patients, health and territories. French Official Journal, Law No. 2009-879 July 21, 2009.

16. Decree No. 2010-1229 of October 19, 2010 on telemedicine [Internet]. Journal officiel Français, 2010-1229 Oct 21, 2010. Available on: ELI: https://www.legifrance.gouv.fr/eli/decret/2010/10/19/SASH1011044D/jo/texte

17. Canada. Personal Information Protection and Electronic Documents Act [Internet]. October 1, 2013. Available at: 29   .https://laws-lois.justice.gc.ca/fra/lois/P-8.6/

18. LAWS OF MALAYSIA Act 564 TELEMEDICINE ACT 1997. Jan 1, 2006 p. 11.

19. World Medical Association. World Medical Association Statement on Responsibility, Accountability and Ethical Guidelines in the Practice of Telemedicine [Internet]. WMA; 2018. Available at: https://www.wma.net/fr/policies-post/prise-de-position-de-lamm-sur-les-responsabilites-et-les-directives-ethiques-liees-a-la-pratique-de-la-telemedecine/

20. Haj Salem N, Ouelha D, Gharbaoui M, Saadi S, Ben Khelil M. Forensic aspects of Telemedicine in Tunisia in the context of the Covid-19 pandemic. Tunis Med. 2020;98(06):423-33.

21. Official Printing Office of the Republic of Tunisia. Law n° 2018-43 of July 11, 2018, supplementing Law n° 91-21 of March 13, 1991, relating to the exercise and organization of the profession of physician and dentist. Official Gazette of the Republic of Tunisia July 17, 2018 p. 2422.

22. Official Printing Office of the Republic of Tunisia. Tunisian Penal Code [Internet]. Official Journal of the Tunisian Republic 2015. Available at: www.iort.gov.tn

23. Official Printing Office of the Republic of Tunisia. Code of medical ethics [Internet]. Official Journal of the Tunisian Republic 2018. Available at: www.iort.gov.tn

24. Law No. 83-112 on the general status of State employees, local public authorities and public administrative establishments. Journal Officiel de la République Tunisienne Dec 16, 1983 p. 3214-25.

25. Official Printing Office of the Republic of Tunisia. Organic Law No. 2004-63 of July 27, 2004, on the protection of personal data. Internet]. Official Journal of the Tunisian Republic, 2004-07-30 Jul 27, 2004 p. 1988-97. Available at: https://www.ilo.org/dyn/natlex/natlex4.detail?p_isn=68055&p_lang=fr

26. Draft Organic Law No. 25/2018 [Internet]. Available at: https://majles.marsad.tn/2014/fr/lois/5accf1ef4f24d0075a86fae9/texte

27. Official Journal of the European Union. REGULATION (EU) 2016/679 OF THE EUROPEAN PARLIAMENT AND OF THE COUNCIL of 27 April 2016 on the protection of individuals with regard to the processing of personal data and on the free movement of such data and repealing Directive 95/46/EC (General Data Protection Regulation) [Internet]. Apr 27, 2016. Available at: http://data.europa.eu/eli/reg/2016/679/oj

28. U.S. Department of Health & Human Services. Summary of the HIPAA Privacy Rule [Internet]. 2008. Disponible sur: https://www.Health Insurance Portability and Accountability Acthhs.gov/hipaa/for-professionals/privacy/laws-regulations/index.html

29. Official Gazette of the Tunisian Republic. Decree 81-1634 of November 30, 1981 on the general internal regulations of hospitals. JORT n°77 dec 4, 1981 p. 2831.

30. Lacour S. From medical confidentiality to electronic health records. Legal considerations on the protection of health data. Medicine Law. June 2016;2016(138):62-9.

31. Collège des médecins du Québec. Medicine, Telemedicine and Information and Communication Technologies. Canada: Collège des médecins du Québec; 2015 Feb.

32. Quantin C, Allaert FA, Auverlot B, Rialle V. Safety, legal and ethical aspects of computerized health data. In: Informatique médicale, e-Santé. Springer-Verlag. Paris: Springer; 2013.

33. General Management of the Healthcare Supply in France. Guide méthodologique pour l'élaboration du programme régional de télémédecine [Internet]. France: Ministère du travail, de l'emploi et de la Santé; 2012 May [cited 20 Dec 2020] p. 116. Available at: https://solidarites-sante.gouv.fr/IMG/pdf/guide_methhodologique_elaboration_programme_regional_telemedecine.pdf

34.   Alami H, Gagnon M-P, Fortin J-P, Kouri RP. La télémédecine au Québec : état de la situation des considérations légales, juridiques et déontologiques. Eur Res Telemed Rech Eur En Telemédecine. June 2015;4(2):33-43.

35.   High Authority of Health. Quality and safety of teleconsultation and téléexpertise : Guide to good practice [Internet]. France: HAS; 2019 May p. 28. Available at: https://www.has-sante.fr/upload/docs/application/pdf/2019-07/guide_teleconsultation_et_teleexpertise.pdf

36.   Beauchamp TL, Childress JF. Principles of biomedical ethics. Eighth edition. New York: Oxford University Press; 2019.

37.   Béranger J. La valeur éthique de la donnée de santé à caractère personnel : vers un nouveau paradigme de l'écosystème médical dématérialisé. Sci Société. 1 Dec 2015;(95):91-105.

38.   Tran V-T, Riveros C, Ravaud P. Patients' views of wearable devices and AI in healthcare: findings from the ComPaRe e-cohort. Npj Digit Med. déc 2019;2(1):53.

39.   Tang PC, Ash JS, Bates DW, Overhage JM, Sands DZ. Personal Health Records: Definitions, Benefits, and Strategies for Overcoming Barriers to Adoption. J Am Med Inform Assoc. 1 mars 2006;13(2):121-6.

40.   Sharpe VA. Privacy and security for electronic health records. Hastings Cent Rep. déc 2005;35(6):49.

41.   Ward L, Innes M. Electronic medical summaries in general practice--considering the patient's contribution. Br J Gen Pract J R Coll Gen Pract. avr 2003;53(489):293-7.

42.   Kluge E-HW. Security and privacy of EHR systems--ethical, social and legal requirements. Stud Health Technol Inform. 2003;96:121-7.

43.   Powell J, Fitton R, Fitton C. Sharing electronic health records: the patient view. J Innov Health Inform. 1 mars 2006;14(1):55-7.

44.   Pyper C, Amery J, Watson M, Crook C. Access to electronic health records in primary care-a survey of patients' views. Med Sci Monit Int Med J Exp Clin Res. nov 2004;10(11):SR17-22.

45.   Hall SE, D'Arcy C, Holman J, Finn J, Semmens JB. Improving the evidence base for promoting quality and equity of surgical care using population-based linkage of administrative health records. Int J Qual Health Care. 1 oct 2005;17(5):415-20.

46.   Chang BL, Bakken S, Brown SS, Houston TK, Kreps GL, Kukafka R, et al. Bridging the Digital Divide: Reaching Vulnerable Populations. J Am Med Inform Assoc. nov 2004;11(6):448-57.

47.   West DM, Miller EA. The Digital Divide in Public E-Health: Barriers to Accessibility and Privacy in State Health Department Websites. J Health Care Poor Underserved. 2006;17(3):652-67.

48.   Kaiser Family Foundation. e-Health and the Elderly: How Seniors Use the Internet for Health Information [Internet]. 2005 janv p. 44. Disponible sur: https://www.kff.org/medicare/poll-finding/e-health-and-the-elderly-how-seniors/

49.   Voelker R. Seniors Seeking Health Information Need Help Crossing "Digital Divide". JAMA. 16 mars 2005;293(11):1310.

50.   Brodie M, Flournoy RE, Altman DE, Blendon RJ, Benson JM, Rosenbaum MD. Health Information, The Internet, And The Digital Divide: Despite recent improvements, Americans' access to the Internet-and to the growing body of health information there-remains uneven. Health Aff (Millwood). nov 2000;19(6):255-65.

51.   Layman EJ. Ethical Issues and the Electronic Health Record. Health Care Manag. oct 2020;39(4):150-61.

52.   Wernick AS. Data theft and state law. J AHIMA. Dec 2006;77(10):40-4; quiz 47-8.

53.   Becker C. Technical difficulties. Recent health IT security breaches are unlikely to improve the public's perception about the safety of personal data. Mod Healthc. 20 févr 2006;36(8):6-7, 16, 1.

54.   Privacy Rights Clearinghouse. Chronology of Data Breaches. USA; 2013 déc p. 137.

55.   Brownstein JS, Cassa CA, Mandl KD. No Place to Hide - Reverse Identification of Patients from Published Maps. N Engl J Med. 19 oct 2006;355(16):1741-2.

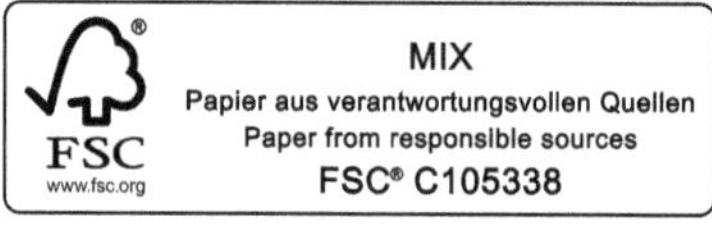

Printed by Books on Demand GmbH, Norderstedt / Germany